ALKALINE DIET

Skyrocket Your Overall Health And Beat Acidity With The Alkaline Diet

KIRSTEN YANG

TABLE OF CONTENT

INTRODUCTION

The food that we take today is totally different from our ancestors and is completely different from what we are so accustomed to these days. How aptly said "We are what we eat." With the advancement of technology, the types of foods we consume made us dragged along.

A view at the grocery store will shock you with aisles and aisles of processed food items and animal products. With the easy availability of fast foods nowadays, there is no difficulty in finding one in our neighborhood.

Fad diets are being partly to blame for introducing a whole new eating habits, this include high-protein diets. In recent years, consumption of animal products and refined food items have increased as more and more people leave out the daily supply of fruits and vegetables in their diets.

It comes as no surprise why, these days, many people are suffering from different types of ailments and allergies such as bone diseases, heart problems and many others. Some health experts link these diseases to the type of foods we eat.

There are certain types of food that disrupts the balance in our body that, during such instances, health problems arise. If only we could modify our eating habits, it's unlikely that prevention of diseases and restoration of health can be achieved.

The theory behind alkaline diet is that because the pH of our body is slightly alkaline, with a normal range of 7.36 to 7.44, our diet should reflect this, and also be slightly alkaline. An unbalanced diet high in acidic foods like animal protein, caffeine, sugar, and processed foods tend to upset this balance.

It can deplete the body of alkaline minerals such as sodium, potassium, magnesium, and calcium, making people vulnerable to chronic and degenerative diseases.

Our internal chemical balance is mainly controlled by our lungs, kidneys, intestines, and skin. For necessary functions to occur, our body must maintain a proper pH.

The measure of the acidity or alkalinity of a substance is called pH. Adequate alkaline reserves are required for optimal adjustment of pH. The body needs oxygen, water, and acid-buffering minerals to accomplish the pH-buffering while quickly removing waste products.

The over-acidification of the body is the underlying cause of all diseases. Soda is probably the most acidic food people consume at a pH of 2.5.

Soda is 50,000 times more acidic than neutral water, and takes 32 glasses of neutral water to balance a glass of soda.

Alkaline food and water should be consumed, in order to provide nutrients the body needs to neutralize acids and toxins from the blood, lymph, and tissues, and at the same time, strengthens the immune and organ systems.

Most vegetables and fruits contain higher amount of alkaline forming elements than other foods. The greater the amount of green foods consumed in the diet, the greater the health benefits achieved.

These plant foods are cleansing and alkalizing to the body, while the refined and processed foods can increase unhealthy levels of acidity and toxins.

But be aware that too much alkaline can also harm you. You must have the proper knowledge of balancing alkaline and acidic foods in your diet.

After ingestion, alkaline food and water is almost immediately neutralized by hydrochloric acid present in the stomach.

The balance between alkaline and acidic foods must be maintained in order for your organs to perform well.

A healthy and balanced diet is more alkaline than acid. Based upon your blood type, the diet should be made up of 60 to 80% alkaline foods and 20 to 40% acidic foods.

Normally, the A and AB blood types require the most alkaline diet while the O and B blood types require more animal products in their diet. But keep in mind; if you're in pain, you're acidic.

CHAPTER 1

WHAT IS ALKALINE DIET AND WHAT FOR?

You have to admit that a diet called the alkaline diet really doesn't have a lot of appeal. It's also called the alkaline acid diet or the acid alkaline diet. This is a diet that emphasizes eating fresh fruits and vegetables, tubers, and nuts and legumes.

The alkaline diet isn't nearly as intimidating as the name makes it sound, although it is very different from what most people eat. It is based on eating few processed plants or animals.

The concept is actually quite simple. You must eat that things that you know are good for your health such as vegetables, and fresh leafy vegetables and you must avoid things that are bad for you such as alcohol, yeast, bad fats, and sugar.

The research is a little more complex than this simple breakdown but the main thing is to maximize the amount of alkaline fruits and vegetables that you eat, as well as alkaline juices and waters.

It emphasizes the 80/20 split of alkaline foods to acidic foods. This is the ratio you should aim for. If it's sounding too complicated, don't worry because it's not. Most of the foods we eat, when they are fully digested will be either alkaline or acidic.

This includes fish, grains, meat, shellfish, poultry, salt, and milk produce acid, all common in the western diet.

While you should eat foods that are more alkaline such as fresh fruits and vegetables, it doesn't always play out that way. As a result we have blood that is slightly alkaline yet still with normal pH levels between 7.35 and 7.45.

This is a diet that's opposite to the high fat, high protein, low carb diets that have become the "in diets." Most have never heard of the alkaline diet or the alkaline acid balance of the body, but holistic doctors and nutritionists are often proponents of this diet because it's believed this type of balance is necessary to stay healthy and prevent the diseases like cancer.

On the other hand many conventional doctors do not believe in or endorse the Alkaline Diet.

Why does one decide to go on an alkaline diet? Many believe chronic disease can be helped by an alkaline diet.

Currently there is not a lot of scientific data to back this particular diet but for the most part just the foods it encourages you eat are healthy foods that are endorsed by most doctors.

This diet might aid those who don't feel well when they eat a diet that's low in carbs or high in protein. It could also benefit those that have stressful lives and who eat too many acidic foods.

THE THEORY OF THE ALKALINE DIET

To keep your body fresh and free of diseases, you have to eat the proper food called alkaline diet or acid alkaline diet. Basically it is a theory that when we eat or consume a food, after several processes like digestion, metabolism and others, it leaves an alkaline residue or acid residue, which determines the acid-alkaline nature of our body.

Alkaline diet theory is based on the fact that the pH of our body is slightly alkaline, that is from 7.35 to 7.45 (in some texts it is 7.36 to 7.44).

Our diet should represent this balance. A disturbance in this balance will cause some severe problems in the body. The nature of liquid whether acidic or alkaline is determined by the pH scale.

It ranges from 0 (very strong acid) to 14 (very strong alkaline). 7 is the neutral point on pH as that of water. A pH below 7 shows acid things, as we go down, becoming strong acidic, and pH above seven represents alkaline products, intensity increasing as we go up to 14.

Medical study of almost every kind has alkaline diet roots although this theory not acknowledge by conventional medical societies.

Diets which contain 60% alkalinity should be used to maintain the balance of the body. One have to use highly alkaline diets (80%) is the balance of his/her body is disturbed by the extensive use of meat, eggs, cream and other acidic foods.

Vegetables, low fat fruits, nuts, tubers fresh citrus and other things should be preferred when talking about alkaline diets. To increase alkalinity in the body, fruits can be used as a good source as mostly fruits are rich in alkaline. A very few number of fruit are acidic.

When eating fruits for this purpose, do not eat canned, or sugared or preserved fruits, because they become highly acidic when preserved due to the use of different chemicals.

Vegetables are highly recommended in alkaline diet theory as they are very good source of making body alkaline.

You will feel weakness rather than power in your body if meat you are eating to gain energy become an acid forming agent in your body, as conventional doctors do not believe in eating vegetables could be useful and persist on eating meat for energy.

Vegetables, especially green vegetables, are very good source of alkaline production and you can use them not only cooked, but vegetables like carrot, cauliflower, tomatoes, and others are used any time you want without even cooking.

They are tasty and provide you with lots of minerals. Minerals like calcium, potassium, and magnesium are the real source of alkaline ash and are very good for the growth and functioning of the body.

Our body is turned from acidic to slightly alkaline when these minerals react with the acid present in out body.

CHAPTER 2

WHY YOU SHOULD ADOPT ALKALINE DIET?

As human beings, we need oxygen to survive; we simply cannot live without it. Now even though you're not a nutritionist, I know you know that oxygen isn't found in cooked or processed foods, nor is it found in meat or cheese.

Oxygen is found in beautiful green chlorophyll. Chlorophyll is the substance in plants that allows them to absorb light from the sun and covert that light into usable energy.

Here's a geeky fact for you; Chlorophyll is chemically related to blood – the only difference being that the main atom is hemoglobin (blood's oxygen transporter) is iron, while in chlorophyll its magnesium.

Chlorophyll contains a powerful blood builder that is said to increase red blood cells, improve circulation, ease inflammation (which we know promotes angiogenesis or cancer cell growth), oxygenates the body and counteracts free radicals. Boy oh boy! This stuff is good! So by feasting on raw fruits, veggies, and dark green leafy we fill our bodies with liquid oxygen, the single most important element keeping us alive.

Here's a little list to help you realize that you are far from being deprived on adopting a more alkaline diet:

Veggies: cucumbers, kale, broccoli, cabbage, cauliflower, celery, spinach, chard, lettuce, parsley, lentil sprouts, onions, garlic, leeks, alflalfa sprouts, broccoli sprouts, green beans, winter squash, sweet potatoes, pak choi, carrots etc

Fruits: avocados, tomatoes, limes, lemons, apples, watermelon, grapes, berries. (Note; lemons, limes and oranges are acidic fruits but actually become alkaline once they are consumed)

There is a whole host of other foods you can eat and I'm not going to lie to you – they don't come in packets or have a shelf life longer than a few days. If it's made in a laboratory or has a shelf life longer than you, do you WANT that in your body?

I could go on for an age about this as there is so much information but the bottom line is that you would be better off if you were to:

Eat raw foods that are living to give you oxygen, enzymes, energy, minerals, vitamins, cancer-fighting phytonutrients etc

Eat foods that are low glycaemic (ie do not send your blood sugar soaring)

If you must eat meat/dairy products then eat organic AND adopt an 80/20 or 70/30 rule where you eat 80/70% raw to 20/30% cooked food. The enzymes in the raw food helps your body to break down the cooked food which is devoid of any enzymes as they get destroyed in the cooking process giving your body more work to do and forces your body to use up the enzymes from it's own reserve.

CHAPTER 3

WHAT ARE THE BENEFITS OF ALKALINE DIETS?

According to nutrition experts, it is an acidic diet that is at least partially responsible for common problems such as premature aging and chronic illness. Health conditions such as arthritis and kidney stones are believed to be linked to diets that are known to generate excessive amounts of acids in the body.

Switching to a low-acid diet is believed to be capable of increasing energy, reducing mucus, relieving symptoms of irritability and anxiety, and may even lead to fewer headaches and infections. Scientists are now looking into claims that an alkaline diet has the power to prevent bone loss, muscle wasting, urinary tract problems, and kidney stones.

Ask people who follow these diets, and they'll tell you that they're healthier, happier, and more energetic than their counterparts who follow more low-carb diets.

Plenty of people have found that their own health issues have either decreased dramatically or been completely eliminated once they adopted alkaline diets. Losing weight is also an important perk for those who incorporate whole foods into their lifestyles.

HOW TO GET THE MOST OUT OF AN ALKALINE DIET

It can be helpful to refer to a list of specific foods, but generally you should attempt to eat an abundance of fresh fruits and vegetables every day. Salads are always a good choice.

Make sure to drink lots of water, vegetable juice, or herbal teas. Avoid processed foods, fried foods, chocolates, foods that contain added sugars, and junk foods.

Instead of adding sugar or salt to the foods you cook, try using healthy and flavorful herbs and spices.

Last but not least, keep in mind that if you overcook your foods, you will be losing much of the nutritional value.

CHAPTER 4

UNDERSTANDING ACID-ALKALINE BALANCE

Health is truly a balance among all the systems of the body. The cells of our body are so interconnected that when you improve the balance of any one system, it improves the balance and vitality of the rest of the organ systems.

For example, improving cardiovascular health improves digestive function. Improving the function of the nervous system will improve the lymphatic system, and possibly most important, when you improve the acid/alkaline balance of the body, you simultaneously improve every other system in the body at the same time.

Finding balance begins in our bloodstream, as does repairing injuries, reducing inflammation, burning fat, building strong bones (reversing osteoporosis), and the increase of energy and vitality.

ALKALINE DIET

In order to function properly, the blood and other body fluids must maintain a very narrow acid/alkaline balance, which is measured by the pH factor (potential hydrogen). pH ranges from 0-14 (very acidic to very alkaline). A pH below 7.0 is acid and above 7 is alkaline. Keep in mind when and if you test your pH that there is a tenfold difference between each number. For example, a pH of 5.0 is 10 times more acidic than a pH of 6.0

Blood pH does not shift easily. The pH of our blood is between 7.25-7.45, and if the blood's pH falls below or above that range, the body cannot function properly.

A tremendous amount of energy is expended to maintain pH levels, all the while pulling from the body's alkaline mineral reserves, causing deficiencies and health disorders.

When we maintain proper pH levels, injuries heal faster and health challenges improve more quickly because the body is oxygenated and therefore can detoxify and heal itself.

If cells are energized in this way, we develop a strong immunity to diseases and a significantly lower propensity for cancer.

The best way to maintain optimal pH levels and optimal vitality is through what we eat and drink and how we react to stress. For the diet, if you follow an 80/20 rule, 80% alkaline forming foods and 20% acid, you should experience all the benefits that a body balance has to offer.

Have a look at the following lists to see which foods do what and where you might be able to increase your alkaline-forming foods. Keep in mind that the foods must be organic because ALL pesticides are very acidic.

ALKALINE FORMING FOODS

DAIRY: acidophilus, whey, kefir/yogurt

FRUITS: apples, apricots, avocados, bananas, berries, cantaloupes, cherries, currants, dates, figs, grapes, grapefruits, guavas, lemons, limes, mangoes, melons, nectarines, oranges, papayas, passion fruits, peaches, pears, persimmons, pineapples, raisins, strawberries, tangerines

VEGGIES: bamboo shoots, green beans, lima beans, string beans, sprouts, beets, broccoli, cabbage, carrots, celery, cauliflower, chard, chicory, chives, collard greens, cucumber, dandelion greens, dill, dulse, eggplant, endive, escarole, kale, garlic, leeks, legumes, lettuce, okra, onions, parsley, parsnips, sweet potato/yam, bell peppers, white potatoes, pumpkin, radish, rutabaga, turnips, watercress

MEAT: No meat is alkaline

NUTS: almonds, chestnuts, coconuts

MISC: ginger, honey, kelp, alfalfa, clover, mint, sage, green tea, quinoa, flaxseed, pumpkin seeds, all seaweed/sea veggies

MINERALS: calcium, magnesium, potassium, manganese

ACIDIFYING FOODS

GRAINS: all white flour products, buckwheat, wheat, corn, barley, oats, rye

DAIRY: butter, eggs, cheese, cottage cheese, cream, ice cream, custards, milk

FRUITS: jams/anything preserved, cranberries, pomegranates, olives

VEGGIES: artichokes, asparagus, garbanzo beans

MEAT: All

NUTS: peanuts, pistachios, walnuts, macadamia

MISC: alcohol, brine, coffee, cocoa/chocolate, candy, many dressings (because of the vinegar), drugs, jams/jellies, mayo, some spices, soda, lack of sleep, stress, worry

TESTING YOUR PH BALANCE

Mild fluctuations inside your body's pH level are routine, which is why you need to use one of many ways available to check your pH level to gain a clear idea of your overall health.

Just like a pool, your body is constructed of water so it is important for you to keep a well-balanced pH and the best way to do so is by determining the status of your system's pH.

By monitoring your pH level over a period of time, you'll be able to note any patterns of acidity or alkalinity levels within your body and so you know you need to find a remedy to improve this imbalance. Should you be looking for methods to test your pH level, here are three ways to start testing it.

TAKE A BLOOD TEST

Probably the most efficient way to find out what your pH level is taking a blood sample test from a physician. The phlebologist then conducts a live cell microscopy to obtain your system's pH level. The blood of a healthy human being is supposed to maintain a pH level ranging from 7.35 to 7.45. Any value below or over this range may have a detrimental impact on your health.

Though choosing a blood test is the most accurate way to determine your pH, it can be an expensive and time-consuming activity. Thus, it isn't the best choice if you are planning to observe your pH level over a given time period.

MEASURE YOUR SALIVA

Our recommendation is that you complete the saliva test each morning immediately after getting up and before eating anything or brushing your teeth. Begin with swallowing all of the saliva in your mouth. Now draft fresh saliva and swallow.

Do this two more times as you prepare your plastic or paper strip. When you draw-up saliva for your third time, spit it on the strip and immediately pay attention to the color of the strip and its particular value (intensity) on the color chart, matching these colors will help you to discover the pH value.

As outlined by medical professionals, the optimum saliva pH after awakening should range between 6.2 to 6.8. This value then moves up towards alkaline levels of (seven.two to seven.four) in daytime.

The one down side to this method is that saliva's pH can be altered by the meal you'd had ahead of the test. Which is the main reason you need to make sure to do the test first thing? It also needs to be noted that even though the paper strip is not toxic, it is advisable to never put it in your mouth.

FINALLY: DO A URINE TEST

The urine test is probably one of the best ways to to find out your pH level particularly if you require a somewhat accurate reading.

Upon awakening, and you are headed for your first "short-call" of the day, wait until you are halfway done then quickly wet your pH test strip (paper or plastic) in the stream of urine and immediately compare the color on the strip to the color on the pH color chart.

To get accurate results, your observation speed can play a big role. This is because pHydrion (the compound used to create the test paper strips) enhances evaporation and if you delay, the color may change resulting in biased results. The optimum urine pH should include 6.2 and 6.8.

In conclusion, you must understand that taking only one pH test isn't enough to conclude what ones' body's pH level is. Various factors such as stress, the food you eat, and also your day to day activities affect your pH levels.

Therefore, it is advisable to use any of the aforementioned methods to test your pH level. You should test several times each day for at least 4 days just to make certain.

CHAPTER 5

ALKALINE FOODS TO EAT AND THOSE TO AVOID

It is essential to maintain a balance in life in all aspects of living. Too much of a good thing can be bad too. The optimum ratio of alkaline and acid ash is said to be 80 % to 20%. If one can maintain this level it would not only rejuvenate his health and youth but also guard against various diseases. To be able to try and achieve this ratio one has to learn about the various types of Acid Alkaline food.

Acid Alkaline foods can be chosen quite simply if a foods nature is known. The various types of foods that are alkaline are mostly fruits and vegetables. Figs have a very high alkaline content in them. That is one of the reasons why it is recommended for people with health problems. Even Banana's help in healing for the same reason.

Garlic is a great healer and also an alkalizing vegetable. Broccoli, cabbage, peas, sprouts and mostly all vegetables are alkalizing foods. Those of us who want to consume sweet things while trying to maintain their alkaline ash levels should consider using stevia since it is an alkalizing sweetener as opposed to sugar.

Apart from cranberries all other fruits also are alkaline in nature. Cranberries are acid ash producing fruits and should not be consumed too much.

For all those meat lovers acid alkaline food charts can really help keep a balance between healthy eating as well as tasty eating. Avoiding red meat and fish, oysters, pork and so on can bring down the acidic ash in one's body.

On the other hand chicken breast is alkalizing food and so are eggs. On the acid alkaline food chats one can clearly see why vegetarianism is getting so popular today. Vegetarians consume a lot of fruits and vegetable so their alkaline ash is higher than their acidic ash. Milk though is not a good bet for those who need to keep their alkaline acid food balance maintained. Even Soymilk is acidifying.

One of the most important ingredients of an acid alkaline food balance is mineral water. Water not only cleanses our system but also reduces the acidic ash levels in our body.

Acid alkaline foods are not acidic or alkaline in their essence. Like say citrus foods are acidic but when consumed they have an alkalizing effect on the urine Ph.

Foods that have an acidic effect on the urine ph are said to be acidic as opposed to the ones that have an alkalizing effect on the urine ph.

The ratio of 4 is to 1 can be maintained easily if acid alkaline foods are consumed in the same ratio.

The kinds of food one eats can affect the body's pH balance. The body is more alkaline as opposed to acidic. One should therefore eat foods that alkalinize after metabolism. That is to say they leave alkaline mineral residues which the body uses in its various functions.

In a nutshell, maintaining an alkaline diet will prevent your body from accumulating metabolic acidity, which is responsible for autoimmune and degenerative diseases.

Alkaline foods are natural, usually green leafy vegetables, nuts, seeds, some types of fruits and healthy oils.

In the next chapter I selected the easiest and more tasty alkaline food recipes you can adopt that will help you attain optimum health.

CHAPTER 6

ALKALINE RECIPES

CHAI-INFUSED VANILLA QUINOA PORRIDGE

There are few more practical and popular brekkies than porridge to set you up with a warming and nourishing start to the day. Oats are a good source of nutrients, including plenty of fibre and complex carbs, to help keep you feeling full right up until lunch. It's well known that a decent breakfast helps to improve your mood and concentration levels, and reduces the likelihood of you reaching for a croissant, pastry or chocolate biscuit by 11am!

Serves: 2

Preparation Time: 8 Minutes

INGREDIENTS:

1 cup of dry quinoa (pref organic)

2 cups of water (pref alkaline)

1 sticks of cinnamon (or 1/2 teaspoon)

1 1/2 teaspoons ground ginger or 1 inch piece of fresh root ginger finely grated

1/2 teaspoon ground nutmeg (pref fresh grated)

1/2 cup of coconut cream or milk (depending on how creamy you want it)

1/2 lemon skin grated (or lime)

1 vanilla bean pod or vanilla essence

Sprinkle (half a handful) of assorted nuts and seeds to your liking

Optional: coconut yoghurt

Optional: cloves, ground

Optional: 1 grated apple (if transitioning)

INSTRUCTIONS

- First prepare the quinoa to the packet instructions OR follow the excellent advice on cooking light fluffy quinoa here at The Kitchen

- Once the quinoa is cooked and drained, add it back to the saucepan and stir in the chai spices (cinnamon, ginger, nutmeg and cloves if you've done them in a pestle and mortar) and add the coconut cream or milk and throw in the scraped out vanilla pod (or add the drop or two of vanilla essence).

- You can pick either the milk or cream depending on how creamy and thick you want it.

- When it's ready, grate in the apple if you're using it – right at the end.

- Warm through and then serve in a big bowl. To serve, add the lemon rind grated onto the top and sprinkle with extra ground cinnamon. Finally throw on the seeds and nuts (I recommend sesame seeds with this especially).

As an indulgent extra, you can also serve with a dollop of coconut yoghurt, which is alkaline and JUST DELICIOUS!

Eat while it's hot!

NUTRITIONAL SUMMARY

This food is very low in Cholesterol and Sodium. It is also a good source of Magnesium, Copper and Manganese.

Alkaline Rating: Neutral

ALKALISING BEAN SALSA BREAKFAST

A warm and filling alkaline breakfast. Great for setting you up for the day.

Serves: 2

Preparation time: 15 minutes

INGREDIENTS:

- 1 can of haricot beans (pref. organic)
- 4 spring onions
- 6 cherry tomatoes
- 1 handful of basil
- 2 handfuls of spinach
- 2 cloves of garlic
- 1 avocado
- ½ lemon
- Olive oil
- Himalayan salt & black pepper

INSTRUCTIONS

- Roughly chop the spring onions, halve the cherry tomatoes, and finely chop the garlic. Now, in a reasonably sized frying pan, bring a little water to the boil (maybe 50ml or less) and 'steam fry' the garlic for one minute. Now throw in the cherry tomatoes, haricot beans and spring onions until everything softens.

- Next add the basil and spinach until it is wilted and season with Himalayan salt and black pepper.

- While this is cooking prepare a side salad and halve the avocado and voila.

- Serve the bean salsa mix with salad and the halved avocado, with lemon and olive oil drizzled all over

NUTRITIONAL SUMMARY

This food is very low in Cholesterol. It is also a good source of Dietary Fiber, Vitamin A, Vitamin C, Folate and Manganese, and a very good source of Vitamin K.

Alkaline Rating: Highly Alkaline

CHICKPEA KALE MASH

Have you ever thought about making a delicious mash without using potatoes and making it a bit more interesting? This recipe is absolutely delicious and uses very healthy and highly alkaline ingredients like kale, garlic and chickpeas.

This mash has got an abundance of different flavours given by the thyme and shallots. You can serve this as a main course or as a side dish with fresh fish.

Serves: 2

Preparation time: 15 minutes

INGREDIENTS:

- 3 tbsp garlic, cut into small pieces

- 1 shallot, cut into small pieces

- 1 bunch kale

- 400g fresh chickpeas (cooked per instructions)

- 2 tbsp Bragg Liquid Aminos (alternative: soy sauce)

- 2 tbsp extra virgin olive oil or coconut oil

- 1/2 tsp of fresh or dried thyme

- Celtic sea salt or Himalayan crystal salt, to taste

INSTRUCTIONS

- Gently fry the shallot and minced garlic in olive oil on medium-high heat until it turns golden brown. Be careful not to burn it, as the garlic becomes bitter tasting otherwise.

- Add the washed and drained kale and stir in the oil, onion and garlic. After the kale has wilted a bit, add the chick peas and cook for about 6 minutes.

- Add the remaining ingredients and stir. Begin mashing the chickpeas with a fork. You can mash them as fine as you like your mash to be.

Enjoy!

NUTRITIONAL SUMMARY

This food is very low in Cholesterol. It is also a good source of Dietary Fiber, Vitamin C and Vitamin B6, and a very good source of Vitamin A, Vitamin K and Manganese.

Alkaline Rating: Highly Alkaline

AVOCADO AND CHICKPEA COMBO

Avocado combined with chickpeas to get some extra fibre and protein!

Serves: 2-3

Preparation Time: 10 Minutes

INGREDIENTS:

- 1 can chickpeas, drained
- 1 ripe avocado
- Himalayan salt & cracked black pepper
- Drizzle of flax oil
- Pinch of cumin
- Optional: herbs of your choice – coriander, basil, parsley

INSTRUCTIONS

- Mix together chickpeas, avocado chunks, salt & pepper along with the cumin and the herbs.

- Mash together leaving some whole chickpeas.

- Drizzle with flax oil, add paprika and serve!

- You can also put this in your veggie & salad wraps for a more filling meal.

NUTRITIONAL SUMMARY

This food is low in Sodium, and very low in Cholesterol. It is also a good source of Protein, Vitamin C, Folate, Calcium, Magnesium and Copper, and a very good source of Vitamin A, Vitamin K and Manganese.

Alkaline Rating: Moderately Alkaline

GLUTEN-FREE SPINACH GARLIC TOFU BURGERS

Who said you can't be healthy eating burgers? With this Gluten-Free Spinach Garlic Tofu Burgers can give you all the taste that you crave and the nutrients that you need.

Serves: 2-4

Preparation Time:

INGREDIENTS:

- 16 ounces frozen spinach (organic), thawed
- 15 ounces firm tofu
- 3/4 cup gluten free rolled oats
- 1 medium onion, chopped
- 3-4 big cloves garlic, minced
- 1/4 cup LSA mix
- 1 tablespoon paprika
- Himalayan salt and pepper to taste
- 1 teaspoon cumin
- 1/4 cup coconut oil
- Optional: dash of Bragg Liquid Amino

INSTRUCTIONS

- Crumble tofu, and mix all ingredients together in bowl. Allow to sit a few minutes so oats can absorb some of the liquid from the spinach.

- Add a little water if your mixture isn't wet enough to hold together. Add the Bragg if desired.

- Make patties with your hands and fry with a little coconut oil. Cook for 6-10 minutes on each side, turning carefully. Serve with a nice big salad!

Nutritional Summary

This food is low in Sodium, and very low in Cholesterol. It is also a good source of Protein, Vitamin C, Folate, Calcium, Magnesium and Copper, and a very good source of Vitamin A, Vitamin K and Manganese.

Alkaline Rating: Moderately Alkaline

DELICIOUS LEMON PASTA

It is alkaline, filling, delicious and very, very quick.

Serves: 2

INGREDIENTS:

- Spelt pasta (enough for 2)
- 1 small broccoli head
- Handful of peas
- 2 garlic cloves
- 1 small courgette
- 1 tomato
- 1/2 red onion
- 2 handfuls of rocket and/or spinach (and any other greens)
- Juice of 1 lemon
- 1 teaspoon of coconut oil
- Drizzle of olive oil
- Himalayan salt & black pepper to taste

INSTRUCTIONS

- Firstly, get the pasta on the go. Then chop all of the greens to a size and shape you like and very lightly fry the broccoli, peas, garlic, red onion and courgette in the coconut oil.

- Once the pasta is ready, drain and put into the pan with the greens, adds the chopped tomato and rocket and stir in the lemon.

- When you're ready to serve, put it all in a bowl and drizzle with olive oil.

Optional: I love chillis so I usually add some at the end. Nice, fresh and hot!

NUTRITIONAL SUMMARY

This food is very low in Cholesterol and Sodium. It is also a good source of Vitamin C, and a very good source of Vitamin K.

Alkaline Rating: Moderately Alkaline

CREAMY COURGETTE PASTA

A fully alkaline and raw pasta dish

Servings: 4

INGREDIENTS:

- 1 Zucchini (courgette)
- 1 Bag of Rocket (arugula)
- 1/2 Red Onion
- 1 Bunch Asparagus
- 12 Basil Leaves
- 4 Tomatoes
- 2 Cloves Garlic
- 4 Servings of Spelt or Vegetable Pasta
- Olive Oil
- Optional Udo's for the Sauce

INSTRUCTIONS

- Start by getting the pasta boiling, once it is ready, remove from the heat and drain to ensure it doesn't go sticky or soggy. Drizzle it with olive oil if it looks like it might stick together and form one giant pasta shape.

- While this is bubbling away, finely dice the red onion and chop the tomato into chunks. Put these to one side with a few handfuls of rocket.

- Now it is time to prepare the sauce – so put 1 chopped up zucchini/courgette, the remaining rocket, the basil and the garlic into a blender with a good drizzle of olive or Udo's oil and blend until it becomes a thick, light green sauce. Salt and pepper to taste.

- Now, stir the sauce in with the pasta (lightly warm if you like, but don't cook!), put into bowls, top with the tomato, red onion and rocket and voila.

Totally raw, alkaline, filling pasta! Brilliant!

NUTRITIONAL SUMMARY

This food is low in Saturated Fat, and very low in Sodium. It is also a good source of Folate and Manganese, and a very good source of Vitamin A, Vitamin C and Vitamin K.

Alkaline Rating: Moderately Alkaline

CLEANSING CHILI-LIME STIR 'FRY'

This is a 100% healthy, alkalizing and delicious recipe with many cleansing ingredients.

The ingredients below taste great – but you can use any greens you have available. Kale works really well!

Serves: 2

INGREDIENTS:

- Pak-Choi
- Carrots
- Mange-Tout/Sugar Snap Peas
- Beansprouts
- Broccoli
- Cabbage (red or green)
- Courgette (Zucchini)
- Fresh Lime Juice
- Chili
- Coriander

- Vegetable Boullion

- Brown Basmati Rice/Wild Rice

INSTRUCTIONS

- Firstly, pulp the coriander with a pestle and mortar along with the finely chopped chili, adding lime juice as you go to make a dressing/sauce. Then set aside to infuse.

- Now chop all of the vegetables fairly finely (so that they will cook quickly). Steam these until they are only just cooked (still a little crunchy).

- Now place all ingredients on a bed of fluffy, steamed rice and cover with the coriander and lime-chili sauce.

Serve, piping hot with a smile.

The beauty of this is it's simplicity. Optionally you can steam fry the vegetables in a vegetable boullion stock if you do not have a steamer.

Another option is to have prawns with this (if you are into seafood).

I have not included quantities as it is probably best to find your own way. Also, of course, feel free to just use whatever vegetables you have available to you.

NUTRITIONAL SUMMARY

This food is very low in Saturated Fat and Cholesterol. It is also a good source of Dietary Fiber, Thiamin, Riboflavin, Vitamin B6, Iron, Magnesium, Phosphorus and Potassium, and a very good source of Vitamin A, Vitamin C, Vitamin K, Folate and Manganese.

ENERGISE POWER MEAL

Here is our Energize Power Meal. It is delicious, filling and only requires about 10 minutes to make! It is vibrant, colorful and packed with anti-oxidants!

Serves: 2

Preparation Time: 10 Minutes

INGREDIENTS:

- 1/4 Red cabbage thinly sliced

- 2 Handfuls of spinach leaves

- 2 Vine-ripened tomatoes, sliced

- 1/2 red onion, diced

- 4 spring onions, thinly sliced/shredded

- 1/2 cucumber, cut into thin matchsticks

- 1 carrot, cut into thin matchsticks or spiralised

- 1/2 broccoli, chopped small

- Handful of beansprouts

- 1 serving of soba noodles

- 1 handful of coriander leaves

- Juice of 1 lime

- Bragg Liquid Aminos/Soy Sauce

Optional: handful of alfalfa sprouts

INSTRUCTIONS

- Tear the coriander and squeeze the lime juice over it to marinate a little.

- Slice everything and prepare the soba noodles.

- Mix together in a big salad bowl with the Bragg or soy sauce and eat!

- This meal is 90% raw, but with warmth and substance from the noodles.

If you want to keep this meal alkaline then use Bragg because soy sauce is acidifying in the body.

NUTRITIONAL SUMMARY

This food is very low in Saturated Fat and Cholesterol. It is also a good source of Dietary Fiber, Thiamin, Vitamin B6, Folate, Magnesium and Potassium, and a very good source of Vitamin A, Vitamin C, Vitamin K and Manganese.

CARROTS, PEAS AND BROCCOLI IN COCONUT CURRY SAUCE

The broccoli, carrots and peas together with the coconut milk and curry powder give this dish an abundance of flavours.

Apart from the great taste, the broccoli, peas and carrots are also very healthy and alkaline, as between them they contain high levels of Vitamin C, dietary fiber, antioxidants and minerals.

We hope You enjoy this tasty curry as much as we do and feel free to mix it up with other vegetables!

Serves: 4

Preparation Time: 30 mins

INGREDIENTS:

- 500g broccoli
- 400g carrots
- 200g peas, fresh or frozen
- 2 medium sized onions
- 3 garlic cloves
- 200ml coconut milk (unsweetened)
- 200ml yeast-free vegetable stock

- 1 lemon (unwaxed)

- 2 tbsp coconut oil

- 2 tsp curry powder

- Optional: Himalayan crystal salt or celtic sea salt

- Freshly ground black pepper

INSTRUCTIONS

- Peel the onions and cut into small pieces.

- Peel the garlic cloves and chop into fine pieces.

- Wash and drain the broccoli and carrots. Separate the broccoli florets from the stem and cut the carrots into thin slices.

- Heat 2 tbs of oil in a large frying pan. Gently fry the onion, garlic and curry powder and shortly roast.

- Add the broccoli and carrots, season with a little bit of salt and briefly fry. Pour in the coconut milk and stock, season with 1/2 tsp grated lemon peel and cover the pan with a lid. Gently cook for about 12 minutes.

- Season the curry with salt, pepper, 1 tbsp lemon juice and curry powder. Quickly bring back to boil and then serve.

NUTRITIONAL SUMMARY

This food is low in Sodium, and very low in Cholesterol. It is also a good source of Dietary Fiber, Folate and Manganese, and a very good source of Vitamin A, Vitamin C and Vitamin K.

ALKALISING CATALAN STEW!

Delicious, warm, filling stew!

Serves: 4

Preparation time: 30 min

INGREDIENTS:

- 6 tbsp olive oil
- 1 large Spanish onion, chopped
- 2 fennel bulbs, chopped
- 1 red chilli, finely chopped
- 1 tsp fennel seeds, ground
- 2 cloves new season garlic, crushed
- ½tsp sweet paprika powder
- 1 tbsp fresh thyme leaves
- 1 tsp saffron strands (optional)
- 3 fresh bay leaves

- 1 tin plum tomatoes

- 250ml/3½ fl oz fish stock or water

- 650g/1 lb 7 oz firm white fish (bream, pollock, cod, monkfish), filleted or Tofu

- 100g/3½ oz toasted almonds, ground

- 1 lemon, cut into wedges

- Quinoa and spring greens

INSTRUCTIONS

- Heat some water in a large pan and steam fry the onions, fennel, chilli, ground fennel seeds and garlic for a few minutes.

- Add the paprika, thyme, saffron, bay leaves and tomatoes and cook until reduced to a thickish sauce.

- Add the fish stock (or water) and bring to a simmer.

- Put the fish pieces/tofu into the stew and stir in the almonds.

- Heat for a minute or two and serve with seasonal greens, quinoa and wedges of lemon.

NUTRITIONAL SUMMARY

This food is low in Sodium, and very low in Cholesterol. It is also a good source of Vitamin C, Calcium and Manganese.

ALKALISING MINESTRONE

Minestrone packed with goodness!

Serves: 2

Preparation Time: 30 Minutes

INGREDIENTS:

- 1/2 cup of eggplant (aubergine)
- 1/2 cup of sweet potato
- 1/2 cup of zucchini (courgette)
- 1/2 cup of carrot
- 1/4 red onion
- 2 cloves of garlic
- 1/2 cup of beans (navy, kidney etc)
- 1 tbsp coconut oil
- 1 cup of vegetable stock
- 1 handful of basil

- 1 cup of tomato juice (fresh or bought)
- Himalayan salt & black pepper

INSTRUCTIONS

- Wash and dice the potato, aubergine and courgette and chop the carrot and onion.

- In a large saucepan, gently sauté these ingredients in the coconut oil for about 2 minutes.

- Add the beans, stock and tomato juice

- Simmer for just 8-10 minutes.

- Stir in the basil and season to taste

NUTRITIONAL FACTS

Each serving contains the following RDA%'s:

- Protein: 10%

- Vitamin A: 322%

- Vitamin C: 114%

- Vitamin E: 10%

- Vitamin K: 624%

- Riboflavin: 11%

- Vitamin B6: 12%

- Folate: 57%

- Calcium: 10%

- Iron: 15%

- Magnesium: 20%

- Potassium: 24%

- Manganase: 58%

- Dietary Fibre: 11%

This food is low in Sodium, and very low in Cholesterol. It is also a good source of Dietary Fiber, Vitamin K, Vitamin B6, Potassium and Manganese, and a very good source of Vitamin A and Vitamin C.

ALKALISING VEGETABLE BEAN SOUP

The core ingredients of this Tuscan soup are green vegetables and beans, which make this soup not only delicious but also highly nutritious and alkaline!

Serves: 2

INGREDIENTS:

- 250g of green vegetables (a selection of green cabbage, spinach and rucola works very well)

- 1 carrot

- 1 celery stick

- 2-3 garlic cloves

- 60g of sprouted bread from the day before (or healthiest alternative)

- 1-2 rosemary twigs

- 4 tbsp olive oil

- 1 litre of yeast-free vegetable stock (organic if possible)

- 1 can of precooked white beans

- 1 red onion

- Celtic Sea Salt or Himalayan Salt

- Freshly ground black pepper

INSTRUCTIONS

- Wash the green vegetables and roughly cut them into pieces. Peel the carrot, wash the celery stick and cut both into strips and then small cube-size pieces. Peel the garlic cloves and cut them into very fine pieces. Cut the sprouted bread into cube-size pieces. Wash the rosemary twigs, take off the needles and cut them into small pieces.

- Gently heat 1 tbsp of the oil in a large pot. Add the carrot, celery and garlic and fry them very briefly in the oil. Stir in the rest of the vegetables together with the rosemary.

- Add the bread and stock and let it heat up. Reduce the heat to medium level and cover the pot with a lid. Cook the vegetables for about 15 minutes until they start to soften.

- Drain the canned beans in a colander and let cold water run over them, until all the liquid from the can has fully drained. Add the beans to the soup and let it cook for about 25 minutes whilst stirring occasionally. The aim is for the soup to thicken! Try the soup and season to taste with salt and pepper.

- You have two options now: either leaves the soup to cool down and gently reheat the next day as the Italians do or peel the onion straight after cooking, halve and cut it into very fine strips. Put the onion strips onto a small plate and put the pot of soup straight onto the dining table. Take as much Ribollita as you like, sprinkle over the onion strips and drizzle over some olive oil.

NUTRITIONAL SUMMARY

This food is low in Saturated Fat, and very low in Cholesterol. It is also a good source of Dietary Fiber, Protein, Vitamin B6, Calcium, Iron, Magnesium and Potassium, and a very good source of Vitamin A, Vitamin C, Vitamin K, Folate and Manganese.

ALKALINE TOM YUM SOUP

Nice and spicy and refreshing at the same time. What more could you ask for.

Serves: 2

Preparation Time: 25 mins

INGREDIENTS:

- 1 stick of lemongrass
- 1-2 red chillis
- 1/2 brown onion cut into large chunks
- Small amount, two small strips of Galangal
- Similar amount of fresh ginger
- 2 Keffir Lime leaves
- 2 cloves of garlic
- 2 Tomatoes quartered
- Handful of coriander

- Bragg Liquid Amino's or Soy Sauce (Bragg is more alkaline)

- 600ml of Vegetable Stock (made with Vegetable Bouillon or yeast-free stock cubes)

As much tofu as you'd like cubed

INSTRUCTIONS

- First, prepare all of the flavors. So chop a few thin strips of ginger and galangal, cut the stem from the chilli and bash it with the flat part of the knife (you don't need to chop), cut the lemongrass into 1.5 inch pieces and bash flat. Bash the garlic and rip the lime leaves into two. You should be salivating at the smell of these flavors by now.

- Now, throw those flavoursome pieces into a large pot with the stock and the onion. Once it has come to the boil add the tofu. Two mins later add the tomato and a minute after that add the coriander and bean sprouts if you fancy, then remove from the heat and serve immediately.

- The soup should be hot and tasty. If you want it sweeter and are happy to be less than 100% alkaline you can add a pinch of brown sugar. Season with salt and pepper.

I love it without the sugar but hey, you might want to take the edge off the chilli!

NUTRITIONAL SUMMARY

This food is very low in Cholesterol and Sodium. It is also a good source of Protein, Vitamin A, Vitamin K, Vitamin B6, Folate, Iron, Magnesium, Phosphorus, Potassium and Copper, and a very good source of Vitamin C, Calcium and Manganese.

TOMATO & AVOCADO ALKALISING SOUP

Delicious served warm or cold!

Serves: 2

INGREDIENTS:

- 5 large ripe (pref vine) tomatoes.
- 1 ripe avocado
- 1 spring onion
- 1/4 cup ground almonds (freshly done yourself, not packet)
- 1 cup broth from Swiss Vegetable Bouillon
- 1/4 teaspoon dill seed
- Dash cayenne pepper
- Himalayan salt & cracked black pepper to taste

INSTRUCTIONS

- Wash and drain all the vegetables. Peel the carrots and cut into slices. Cut the courgettes into thick batons. Dry the spinach leaves and lay them in a shallow serving dish.

- Place the olive oil into a wide oven-proof dish over low heat. Add the carrots and peppers and season with salt and pepper according to taste. Cover the casserole dish and cook gently for about 30 minutes or until the vegetables are tender.

- Stir in the courgettes and, cover again and cook for about another 10 minutes. The courgettes should be tender but still have their colour.

- To serve place the warm salad with all the juices onto the spinach leaves.

TORTILLA SOUP

Filling, Full of Protein and Raw Nutrients.

Serves: 4

Preparation Time: 20 Minutes

INGREDIENTS:

- 500ml of (alkaline) water
- 2 teaspoons of vegetable bouillon or 1 yeast-free vegetable stock cube
- 1 ripe avocado
- 1/2 red capsicum (pepper)
- 1 tomato
- 1/2 bunch of coriander (cilantro)
- 2 large handfuls of spinach
- 2 cloves of garlic
- 1 lime

- 1 corn on the cob (about 4 inches long)

- 1 chili/jalapeno (to your taste)

- Pinch of black pepper and Himalayan (or Celtic Sea) Salt

- 1 sprouted tortilla wrap

INSTRUCTIONS

- Slicing your tortilla into 1cm wide and 5cm long strips and toast under the grill

- Boil the alkaline water in a large saucepan and dissolve the stock cubes/bouillon to make a vegetable broth.

- Dice the peppers/capsicum and tomato and tear the coriander

- Peel and dice the avocado

- Mince the garlic

- Slice the chili/jalepeno to your preference

- Wash and roughly chop the spinach and dry with a tea towel

- Now finally prepare the corn by slicing the kernels from the cob with a sharp knife

- Put everything in the broth and heat through

ALKALINE QUINOA SALAD

Filling, Full of Protein and Raw Nutrients

Serves: 2

Preparation Time: 10 Minutes

INGREDIENTS:

- 15 cherry tomatoes
- 1 serving of quinoa
- 1 carrot
- 1 avocado
- 1 beetroot
- A handful of baby peas
- A handful of basil
- A good pinch of sage leaves
- A pinch of healthy salt (Celtic, Himalayan etc)
- A pinch of black pepper
- A dressing of olive oil with lemon juice

INSTRUCTIONS

- Mix one part quinoa to five parts water, bring to the boil and simmer gently until the water has absorbed

- Steam baby peas gently for a few minutes to cook through and then put aside.

- Grate (or use a spiral slier) the carrot and beetroot into a bowl.

- Slice your avocado as you like and then mix all of this into a large bowl with the herbs

- Chop tomatoes in half, drizzle with olive oil and place under the grill for about 5 minutes

- Mix it all up into a big bowl and dress with the olive oil and lemon juice.

NUTRITIONAL SUMMARY

This food is low in Sodium, and very low in Cholesterol. It is also a good source of Dietary Fiber, Vitamin C, Folate and Manganese, and a very good source of Vitamin A and Vitamin K.

KALE SALAD

A 100% highly alkalising salad - a contrast in flavour and texture of the kale against the soft, sweet tomatoes.

Serves: 2

Preparation Time: 10 Mins

INGREDIENTS:

- 1 Big bunch of Kale
- 2 Carrots
- 2 Handfuls of cherry/baby plum tomatoes
- 1 Lemon, juiced
- ½ Cup soaked pine nuts
- ¼ Cup of sesame seeds
- 1 Medium red onion
- Raw black olives
- 1/4 Cup of Olive/Avocado oil or Udo's Choice
- A pinch of Himalayan Salt

- A Few dashes of Bragg Liquid Aminos or pHlavor

- A Pinch of black pepper

INSTRUCTIONS

- Firstly, shred the kale so that it is nice and fine, grate the carrots and cut the tomatoes in half.

- Slice the onion quite thin and half the olives (make sure there are no seeds in the olives).

- Mix into a large bowl with everything else!

- If you are transitioning you can also add some sun-dried or semi-dried tomatoes, goats cheese etc to this recipe, but to be honest it is delicious enough as it is!

- Enjoy as a main in itself or as a salad alongside your main dish.

NUTRITIONAL SUMMARY

This food is low in Sodium, and very low in Cholesterol. It is also a good source of Dietary Fiber, Magnesium and Copper, and a very good source of Vitamin A, Vitamin C, Vitamin K and Manganese.

SPINACH AND ROAST GARLIC SALAD

This salad contains both spinach and roast garlic, which are both packed with nutrients and are highly alkalising.

Spinach is such a versatile vegetable as it can be fried, quickly boiled or steamed. It is extremely rich in antioxidants and a great source of vitamin A, vitamin E, vitamin K, vitamin C, manganese, magnesium, iron, folate, zinc just to name a few. Garlic is also one of the oldest known medicinial plants and is known for a myriad of health benefits.

Serves: 4

Preparation Time:

INGREDIENTS:

- 500g baby spinach leaves, washed and drained
- 10 garlic cloves, unpeeled
- ca 40g pine nuts, lightly toasted
- Fresh juice of 1/2 lemon
- 4 tbsp extra virgin olive oil
- Celtic sea salt or himalayan crystal salt
- Freshly ground black pepper

INSTRUCTIONS

- Preheat your oven to about 180 Celsius.

- Place the garlic cloves into a roasting dish, add in about 2 tbsp of the oil and bake for about 10-15 minutes until the garlic cloves have turned slightly golden and have started to soften.

- Tip the garlic into a salad bowl. Add the lemon juice, pine nuts, spinach, remaining olive oil and season to taste.

NUTRITIONAL SUMMARY

This food is low in Sodium, and very low in Cholesterol. It is also a good source of Vitamin E (Alpha Tocopherol) and Magnesium, and a very good source of Vitamin A, Vitamin C, Vitamin K, Folate and Manganese.

WARM COURGETTE, RED PEPPER AND SPINACH SALAD

This Mediterranean style salad is not only tasty and flavoursome, but very healthy and nutritious too!

Red peppers, spinach and courgettes are highly alkalising and are also packed with important nutrients. They contain high levels of Vitamin C, A, manganese, folate and potassium.

Serves: 2

Preparation Time:

INGREDIENTS:

- 1 red pepper, de-seeded
- 450 g courgettes
- 300 g fresh baby spinach, washed and drained
- 350 g carrots, cut into slices
- 150 ml extra virgin olive oil
- Himalayan crystal salt or celtic sea salt
- Freshly ground pepper

INSTRUCTIONS

- Wash and drain all the vegetables. Peel the carrots and cut into slices. Cut the courgettes into thick batons. Dry the spinach leaves and lay them in a shallow serving dish.

- Place the olive oil into a wide oven-proof dish over low heat. Add the carrots and peppers and season with salt and pepper according to taste. Cover the casserole dish and cook gently for about 30 minutes or until the vegetables are tender.

- Stir in the courgettes and, cover again and cook for about another 10 minutes. The courgettes should be tender but still have their color.

- To serve place the warm salad with all the juices onto the spinach leaves.

ENERGIZING BEAN HUMMUS

Boost Your Digestive System with Black Bean Hummus

Serves: 2

Preparation Time: 10 Minutes

INGREDIENTS:

- 1 can black beans (200g), rinsed and drained
- 2 teaspoons fresh lemon juice
- 1 small handful of basil leaves
- 1 clove of garlic, crushed
- 1 large pinch of sesame seeds

Optional: red chilli to taste

INSTRUCTIONS

- Process black beans, lemon juice, basil, sesame seeds and garlic, in a food processor, until thick. If it's TOO thick, you can add a little water or tahini (if you have it).

NUTRITIONAL FACTS

Each serving contains the following RDA%'s:

- Molybdenum   129.00 mcg 172.0

- Folate   256.28mcg 64.1

- Fiber   14.96 g 59.8

- Tryptophan   0.18 g 56.2

- Manganese   0.76 mg 38.0

- Protein   15.24 g 30.5

- Magnesium   120.40 mg 30.1

- Vitamin B1   0.42 mg 28.0

- Phosphorus   240.80 mg 24.1

- Iron   3.61 mg 20.1

This food is low in Saturated Fat, and very low in Cholesterol and Sodium. It is also a good source of Protein, Thiamin, Magnesium, Phosphorus, Copper and Manganese, and a very good source of Dietary Fiber and Folate.

ASPARAGUS DELIGHT

Simple and delicious starter or alternatively just place the asparagus on top of a nice healthy salad and put the dressing over both

Serves: 2

INGREDIENTS:

- 12 asparagus stems (bend towards the end and let them snap naturally, a la Jamie Oliver)
- 8 spring onions
- 2 tablespoons melted (avocado) butter
- Grated lemon peel of half a lemon
- Fresh lemon juice of a whole lemon
- Fresh thyme

INSTRUCTIONS

- Lightly steam the asparagus and spring onion together (for about 4 minutes or until as tender as you like – although remember, overcooking removes nutrients!)

- Then, mix together the avocado butter, lemon rind, juice and thyme to make a dressing.

- If it is too zingy, then add some cold-pressed extra virgin olive oil to neutralize the lemon a little.

- Now decoratively stack the asparagus and spring onion and dress. Voila!

NUTRITIONAL SUMMARY

This food is very low in Cholesterol and Sodium. It is also a good source of Vitamin A, Potassium and Copper, and a very good source of Dietary Fiber, Vitamin C, Vitamin K and Folate.

ENERGISE QUICK KALE CHIPS

Delicious, Alkaline & Super Healthy Snack

Serves: 4

Preparation Time: 45 Minutes

INGREDIENTS:

- 1 bunch of kale (cavolo nero works better than curly kale)
- 1 tablespoon of oil (olive or flax works best)
- 1 pinch of Himalayan salt

Optional:

- Dried Chilli Flakes
- 1 tsp of Paprika

INSTRUCTIONS

- Preheat the oven to 200°C / 400°F.

- Rip the kale into chips (about 2-4cm squares).

- Rub and toss the chips in the oil and the salt.

- Spread the chips out on a baking tray and pop them in the oven for up to 10 minutes.

NUTRITIONAL SUMMARY

This food is low in Sodium, and very low in Cholesterol. It is also a good source of Copper, and a very good source of Vitamin A, Vitamin C, Vitamin K and Manganese.

COCONUT CHIA PUDDING

It's an alkaline, delicious dessert you can serve to the family, at a dinner party, you can take it to work in your packed lunch…

And it packs a whole lotta omega 3, fibre, alkaline minerals, vitamins, antioxidants…it's amazing.

There are a couple of not 100% alkaline ingredients in here, but they are outweighed easily by the alkaline ingredients. But they add some delicious flavour and make this a huge hit.

Remember, we're never aiming for perfection, we're aiming to make being healthy a fun, enjoyable and delicious experience for life.

Serves: 4

Preparation Time: 20 Minutes

INGREDIENTS:

- 1 cup of (organic) coconut milk
- 1/4 cup of chia seeds
- 1 date
- 1 cup of coconut yoghurt

- 1 tablespoon of flax seeds, ground, or 1 tablespoon of flax meal

- 1 tsp of sesame seeds

- 1/2 teaspoon of vanilla extract

Toppings for 3 varieties:

- 1 handful of blueberries

- 1 handful of mixed nuts (almonds, macadamia, pistachios, Brazil nuts etc)

- 1 tsp of ground cinnamon

INSTRUCTIONS

- Firstly, sweeten the coconut milk by blending with the date. This little touch of sweetness and flavour from the date makes a huge difference!

- Next combine the coconut milk in a large bowl with chia seeds, vanilla, flaxmeal (ground flax) and sesame seeds.

- Put into the fridge for 20-30 minutes until the chia has expanded.

- To serve, fill a small glass with a layer of coconut yoghurt, followed by the chia mix, then a little extra layer of coconut yoghurt.

- Top with your choice of toppings!

The three varieties I love are:

- Simply with blueberries (a fruit that is very mildly acid forming, but delicious with this mix and the dish is still overall alkaline forming)

- With mixed nuts and cinnamon – yum!

- With fig for a sweeter, more exotic flavor to complement the coconut!

A final variation would be to mix 2 teaspoons of raw cacao powder in with the chia or with the coconut milk (when you blend in the dates) to make it a chocolate chia cream pot!

Enjoy and test it on your family and friends!

It's creamy, delicious and alkaline!

NUTRITIONAL SUMMARY

This food is very low in Cholesterol and Sodium. It is also a good source of Dietary Fiber and Manganese.

ORIGINAL GREEN SMOOTHIE

Delicious Antioxidant-Rich, Green, Alkaline, full of healthy oils and protein!

Serves: 2

Preparation Time: 15 Minutes

INGREDIENTS:

- A handful of Kale
- A handful of Spinach
- 2 Broccoli heads
- 1 Tomato
- A handful of Lettuce
- 1 Avocado
- 1 Cucumber
- 1/2 clove Garlic
- Juice of 1/2 Lemon
- A little water to the texture you like

INSTRUCTIONS

- Blend the avocado, cucumber and lemon juice to form a paste, then add the other ingredients.

- You can blend in a little ice if you prefer it chilled, or add a little chilli.

OPTIONAL: Sweeten it up with some capsicum (pepper).

NUTRITIONAL SUMMARY

This food is low in Sodium, and very low in Cholesterol. It is also a good source of Dietary Fiber, Vitamin B6, Folate, Potassium, Copper and Manganese, and a very good source of Vitamin A, Vitamin C and Vitamin K.

Alkaline Rating: Highly Alkaline

Protein Completeness: Provides 98% of all protein types required

Nutrient Balance: Provides 75% of all nutrients required for optimal health

Glycemic Index: 16 (low)

Weight Loss: 4.5/5

Optimum Health: 5/5

Proven Health Benefits: Antioxidant, Energy, Nervous System, Psychological Function, Blood Health, Immune Health, Hormonal Health, Muscle, Bone, Skin, Eyes, Teeth and Hair!

LIVER CLEANSE RECIPE

This is an excellent liver cleanse recipe that I have adapted from about four or five other liver cleanse recipes that I have tried over the years. I have supercharged it with a few extra ingredients, but have put the main, base ingredients in bold to highlight the essentials.

I would recommend doing this over the weekend, and in the morning. It is particularly effective if you have undertaken some light exercise such as walking or jogging prior to the liver cleanse as this helps to get the toxins moving out of the body and invigorates the lymph system.

After the juice I would also recommend some breathing exercises to help the lymph flow on its way.

Serves: 2

Preparation Time: 10 Minutes

INGREDIENTS:

- 2 large grapefruits

- 4 lemons

- 300ml of alkaline water (or filtered)

- 2 tablespoons of Udo's Choice (or cold pressed flax oil

- 1 teaspoon of acidophilus

- 1-2 cloves of fresh garlic

- 2 inches of fresh root ginger

Optional: a dash of cayenne pepper!

INSTRUCTIONS

- Squeeze the juice of the grapefruit and lemon into a blender

- Next, grate the garlic and the ginger, and then using a garlic press, squeeze this into the juice

- Now add the water, Udo's and acidophilus powder and blend for 30 seconds

- Add more ginger/garlic to taste

This juice contains all of the most potent liver cleansing ingredients, and gives your liver a gentle flush and the opportunity to heal itself. There are no side effects to this drink, apart from a bit of garlic-breath for a while. However, the grapefruit removes most of the odour.

I have also been told that this liver cleanse recipe is the most incredible hangover cure in the world – so it might be worth bearing in mind just for that! It contains everything you would need to cure a hangover (vitamin c, omega 3, probiotics, water, ginger) so I can see how it would work!

NUTRITIONAL SUMMARY

This food is very low in Cholesterol and Sodium. It is also a very good source of Vitamin C. It is a good source of vitamins A, E, K, Thiamin, B6, Folate and the alkaline salts Magnesium and Potassium.

Alkaline Rating: Highly Alkaline

Glycemic Index: 14 (low)

Weight Loss: 3/5

Optimum Health: 3/5

Proven Health Benefits: Antioxidant, Energy, Nervous System, Psychological Function, Blood Health, Immune Health, Hormonal Health, Muscle, Bone, Skin, Eyes, Teeth and Hair!

CONCLUSION

Touted as one of the best diets you can follow, the alkaline diet is more than just quick fix way of eating; it should be a lifestyle and a habit. With promises of helping you lose weight and stave off chronic diseases, its little wonder that thousands of people are so keen to try it.

The secret to eating an alkaline diet is simple: choose to eat foods rich in whole, fresh fruits and vegetables while staying away from animal products and heavily processed ingredients.

Cutting out processed foods and turning towards natural options instead provides a tremendous advantage for your health, and it's sure to keep your body balanced.

If you're ready to take your health more seriously, make a commitment to live an alkaline diet today! You'll be amazed how much better you feel.

Made in the USA
Middletown, DE
26 October 2017